ESSENTIAL GUIDE TO PRURIGO NODULARIS

Understanding, Managing, and Overcoming Prurigo Nodularis: A Comprehensive Guide for Patients and Healthcare Professionals

DR. CASEY LOREN

DISCLAIMER

This book's content is only meant to be used for general informative purposes. Although the author has taken great care to ensure the content is accurate and thorough, no warranties or assurances on the information's accuracy, correctness, or reliability are provided. It is recommended that readers employ their own judgment and discretion when applying any material found in this book to their particular situation.

The information in this book is not intended to replace professional advice, nor is the author an expert in any of the subjects covered. It is recommended that readers consult with experienced professionals regarding any particular issues or concerns.

Any name that may be mentioned or referred in this book does not imply endorsement, recommendation, or relationship on the part of the author with any person, entity, good, website, or association. These references are made only for informational purposes and are not meant to be taken as recommendations or endorsements.

The information contained in this book may cause readers to suffer loss or damage, for which the author disclaims all obligation and accountability. The only people accountable for the decisions and actions taken by readers using the information presented are themselves.

Any names, characters, companies, locations, activities, occasions, and incidents referenced in this book are either made up or the result of the author's imagination. Any likeness to real people, living or dead, or to real things is entirely coincidental.

This book's content may change at any time, without prior notice, according to the author. The onus is on the reader to verify whether there have been any updates or revisions.

The reader accepts the conditions of this disclaimer by reading this book. Please do not read this book or use its contents if you do not agree to these terms.

Table of Contents

CHAPTER 1

A COMPREHENSIVE GUIDE TO PRURIGO NODULARIS

What is Prurigo nodularis and What It Is?

Intensely irritating nodules or pimples appear on the skin of people with prurigo nodularis, a chronic skin ailment. The arms, legs, and trunk are common locations for these nodules, which can range in size and color. Prurigo nodularis is characterized by intense, long-lasting itching that can cause additional skin damage from scratching.

Factors that Can Lead to **Causes**

Several variables may have a role in the development of prurigo nodularis, although the specific cause is yet unknown. Some examples are:

1. **Skin Irritation:** Nodules can develop on the skin as a result of persistent skin rubbing or scratching.

2. Prurigo nodularis can occur in conjunction with other skin disorders such as psoriasis, dermatitis, or eczema.

3. **Neurological Factors:** Prurigo nodularis can occur because of problems or irregularities in the nervous system.

4. Some people may be more likely to develop the illness due to a genetic predisposition.

5. The development of nodules and an increase in itching can be brought on by psychological factors such as stress and anxiety.

Noticeable Indications

Itching that is both severe and persistent is the main sign of prurigo nodularis. There can be further signs:

1. Raised, hard bumps on the skin, which can range in size and color, are known as skin nodules.

2. The skin might become thicker, scaly, or discolored as a result of continuous scratching, which is known as skin damage.

3. **Secondary Infections:** It's more likely that germs may invade skin wounds caused by scratching.

Methods for Diagnosis

Medical history, physical exam, and occasionally skin biopsies are the main components of a prurigo nodularis diagnosis. Additionally, your doctor may want to know how long you've been experiencing itching, what triggers it, and what helps or hurts it.

The Significance of Prompt Identification

To properly manage prurigo nodularis and avoid consequences such as skin infections or increased irritation, early identification is vital. Improved health outcomes and quality of life can result from quick medical attention seeking.

Effects on People's Standard of Living

The severity of Prurigo nodularis can greatly affect a person's standard of living. Feelings of anxiety, sadness, and disturbed sleep may result from persistent itching and discomfort. The skin changes and apparent nodules may also affect one's sense of self-worth and body image.

Ongoing Methods of Treatment

Prurigo nodularis treatment goals include itching relief, inflammation reduction, and skin damage prevention. Some common choices for treatment are:

1. Applying a steroid cream or ointment topically helps alleviate swelling and itching.

2. To regulate the skin's immune response, a doctor may recommend a drug called a topical immunomodulator, such as tacrolimus or pimecrolimus.

3. Oral antihistamines are useful for reducing itching, particularly during the night.

4. It is possible that some individuals may benefit from phototherapy, which involves exposure to ultraviolet radiation (UVB or UVA) under medical supervision.

5. For more serious instances, a doctor may recommend oral corticosteroids, immunosuppressants, or antipruritic drugs.

Prurigo nodularis management presents unique obstacles.

Managing prurigo nodularis can be quite a challenge because the condition is chronic, the itching never goes away, and relapses can happen even after therapy. Medication side effects are another concern for patients, and it may take some trial and error to determine the best course of treatment.

Developments and Research

Research into prurigo nodularis is ongoing to improve treatment choices and understand its underlying causes. The development of novel drugs, the function of the nervous system in itching, and the influence of genes are all areas that need further investigation.

Methods for Coping and Resources for Helping Oneself

Although prurigo nodularis is a challenging condition to live with, there are ways to cope and resources to lean on:

1. **Avoiding Triggers:** When you know certain textiles or environmental variables aggravate your itching, you can try to avoid them.

2. **Skin Care:** Gently caring for your skin, such as using a moisturizer regularly and staying away from harsh soaps, can help alleviate irritation.

3. Counselling, support groups, or therapy can help with the emotional burden of the condition, which is known as psychological support.

4. One way to help those around you understand and cope with prurigo nodularis is to educate them. This includes your loved ones, friends, and healthcare providers.

To sum up, prurigo nodularis is a difficult ailment that causes nodules to form on the skin and severe itching. Management of the disorder and improvement of affected individuals' quality of life require early discovery, thorough treatment approaches, ongoing research, and supporting initiatives.

CHAPTER 2

POPULATION HEALTH AND STATISTICS

The Prurigo Nodularis Epidemic and Its Distribution

A chronic skin ailment known as Prurigo Nodularis (PN) causes extremely irritating nodules or papules, which can greatly impact a person's quality of life and cause a great deal of distress. To better diagnose, treat, and support those affected by PN, it is essential to understand its demographics and epidemiology.

Worldwide Rates of Incidence

The prevalence of PN varies greatly across populations and areas around the world. Although PN is a rare dermatological illness, it is relevant since it affects an estimated 1-5% of the general population. Underdiagnosis, misdiagnosis, and differences in healthcare reporting and access make it difficult to acquire accurate prevalence data.

Distribution by Gender and Age

Although PN can strike at any age, the peak incidence is in the 30–60 age group in adults. Women are slightly more likely to be afflicted than men, suggesting a minor predominance. Hormonal, genetic, or immunological variables may all play a role in explaining this gender gap, but no one knows for sure.

Differences by Region

The frequency and manifestation of PN can vary across different regions. It seems to be more prevalent in areas where particular environmental elements are prevalent or among people who have greater rates of related medical disorders. The detection and reporting of PN cases vary among regions due to factors such as healthcare accessibility and diagnostic tool availability.

Prurigo nodularis and ethnicity

Although people of all races and ethnicities are susceptible to PN, some research has shown that some groups are more likely to acquire the condition or have more severe symptoms. Additional studies are required to determine if these findings are due to environmental or genetic causes and to define the function of ethnicity in PN epidemiology.

Economic and Social Considerations

The management and prevalence of PN can be greatly affected by socioeconomic factors such as income, education, and access to healthcare. There may be more illness load and worse outcomes for those of lower socioeconomic class because they are less likely to have access to timely diagnoses, expert care, and effective therapies.

Medical Issues That May Occur Together

It is common for PN to coexist with other medical issues, such as atopic dermatitis, chronic renal illness, liver disorders, HIV/AIDS, mental disorders, and autoimmune diseases. To properly assess, monitor, and address patients, it is crucial to understand these relationships and any comorbidities that may lead to the development or worsening of PN.

Effects on Age Groups Diverse

The effects of PN varied throughout age groups. As a result of psychological discomfort, scarring, chronic itching, and pain, PN can significantly lower the quality of life in adults. Pediatric dermatology is necessary since PN can manifest differently in children and presents special diagnostic and treatment issues.

Patterns of Occurrence and Prevalence

There isn't a tonne of information on how common or commonplace PN has become, although some studies have shown that the condition is being more recognized and diagnosed recently. Possible causes include heightened knowledge of PN among medical professionals, better methods of diagnosis, and a deeper appreciation for the toll it takes on patients' daily lives.

Problems in Collecting Data

The problem of gathering reliable epidemiological data on PN is heightened by several obstacles. Among these difficulties are insufficient data from population-based studies, inconsistent diagnostic standards, and an absence of standardized disease classification. To get trustworthy epidemiological insights, it is crucial to work on better data-gathering methods and to interact across healthcare systems.

Looking Ahead Outlook

More interdisciplinary collaboration, focused educational initiatives, and individualized therapy approaches are anticipated to be necessary in the future as PN becomes more well-known and research into the condition progresses. To track PN trends, find risk factors, and optimize patient care techniques, longitudinal research and surveys of the general population are essential.

Scientists, dermatologists, public health organizations, and patient advocacy groups must continue to work together to understand the demographics and epidemiology of Prurigo nodularis. We may endeavour to improve outcomes and assistance for persons living with this difficult skin condition by addressing important factors influencing the prevalence, distribution, and impact of PN.

CHAPTER 3

WHAT CAUSES IT AND HOW IT WORKS

The Prurigo Nodularis Essential Guide to Its Causes and Symptoms

A patient's quality of life can be greatly affected by Prurigo Nodularis (PN), a persistent skin disorder marked by extremely irritating nodules. The key to accurate diagnosis and effective therapy is understanding its pathophysiology and etiology. The essentials will be thoroughly covered in this manual.

Prurigo nodularis: What Causes It?

Prurigo nodularis is a complex condition that can have many different causes, such as:

In many cases, PN will coexist with other long-term skin disorders, such as psoriasis or atopic dermatitis.

It may be linked to systemic disorders like HIV, chronic renal disease, liver disease, and others.

- **illnesses of the nervous system**: PN has been associated with peripheral neuropathies and other neurological illnesses, indicating a complicated interaction between the skin and the nervous system.

Important Neurological Elements

Several neurological variables contribute to the onset and maintenance of PN. Some important points are:

- **Neuropathic itch**: If the central or peripheral nervous system is damaged or malfunctioning, it can cause chronic itching. This can be exacerbated by conditions such as diabetes and post-herpetic neuralgia.

- **Sensitization**: When you itch and scratch all the time, you can make your nervous system hypersensitive to things that cause it to itch.

The production of neuropeptides by cutaneous nerve fibers can cause inflammation and the maintenance of itching, a condition known as **neurogenic inflammation**.

** Immunological Processes**

Crucial to PN is the immune system's role:

T-cell activation: PN lesions show signs of elevated T-cell activity, which could indicate an inflammatory response driven by the immune system.

- **Cytokine release**: PN is associated with an increase in inflammatory and itchy cytokines such as IL-31 and IL-4.

An allergic or hypersensitive component is indicated by elevated levels of eosinophils in PN patients, a condition known as **eosinophilia**.

A Family History of a Disease

A person's susceptibility to PN may run in their family:

tend to run in families.

- **Hereditary markers**: Some variations in genes that affect the immune system or the skin's protective barrier may make people more likely to develop PN.

Environment-Related Factors

Factors in the environment can worsen PN:

The presence of allergens, such as dust mites, pet dander, or specific foods, might cause an exacerbation of symptoms.

• **Climate**: Extremely dry and cold temperatures might worsen itchy skin.

- **Living conditions**: PN can be worsened by stress, an unhealthy diet, and an inadequate amount of sleep.

Important Function of Inflammation

At its core, PN is inflammation:

A thickening of the skin and chronic inflammation are the results of persistent scratching.

Lesions are filled with many types of inflammatory cells, such as lymphocytes, eosinophils, and mast cells.

Imbalances in Neurotransmitters

In the pathogenesis of PN, neurotransmitters are involved:

Anxiety disorders may be associated with changes in serotonin levels and the receptors for this neurotransmitter.

Although histamine is known to mediate itching, the exact nature of its function in PN remains unclear.

- **Substance P**: This neuropeptide has a role in the signaling of pain and itching and is found at higher levels in PN lesions.

The Skin's Pathological Alterations

In PN, the skin goes through several abnormal changes:

The thickening of the skin's outer layer as a result of repeated rubbing causes **epidermal hyperplasia**

- Nodules develop in the dermis as a result of increased collagen deposition, a condition known as dermal fibrosis.

- Elevated density of nerve fibers in the afflicted skin regions: **neuroproliferation**.

A Series of Symptoms

PN is characterized by a series of symptoms:

The signature symptom, **intense itching**, which frequently causes psychological distress and sleeplessness.

Hard, itchy nodules develop when itching and scratching continue for an extended period.

*Changes to the skin**: Common changes include hyperpigmentation, lichenification, and excoriations.

New Hypotheses and Future Paths in Research

Novel PN features are currently the subject of research:

- **Microbiome**: The function of the skin's microbiota in PN is a topic of current research.

- **New treatment approaches**: Researchers are looking into biological medicines that target particular immune pathways.

- Additional genetic investigations are being conducted to identify the genes that are linked to PN susceptibility.

- **Neuromodulation**: Investigations into medications and blockers that act on the nervous system are ongoing.

To improve patient outcomes in Prurigo nodularis and create successful treatments, it is vital to understand the complicated interplay of these elements.

CHAPTER 4

CLINICAL SIGNS AND EVALUATION

Nodules and Lesions That Characterise

Plumbago nodularis (PN) is defined by the presence of several hard, dome-shaped nodules that are hyperkeratotic and can be red, pink, or even skin-colored. Lesions with this size range from 1 to 3 centimeters in diameter and are frequently crusted or scaled over. The nodules can merge into bigger plaques. Lesions are symmetrically dispersed and extremely itchy, which can cause severe excoriation and, in rare instances, subsequent infections. These nodules develop and stay because of the constant picking and itching.

The Level of Itching and Itching Patterns

People with PN generally describe the itching, also known as pruritus, as a burning or stinging feeling, and it's constant and intense. It may occur continuously or in spurts, with worsening symptoms on occasion. The level of itching can greatly affect one's quality of life since it often gets in the way of normal activities and sleep. Anxiety and sadness are secondary psychological consequences that patients may experience as a result of persistent and intense itching.

Skin Involvement Distribution

Lesion patterns of PN most commonly show up on the buttocks and trunk, although they can also spread to the extensor surfaces of the limbs, especially the shins and forearms. Lesions on the scalp, palms, and soles are typically not present. One way to distinguish PN from other skin disorders is by looking for symmetrical lesion distribution; another way is to see whether any regions are spared.

Problems with Differential Diagnosis

Many other pruritic dermatoses share symptoms with PN, making a definitive diagnosis difficult. Nodular scabies, cutaneous lymphoma, lichen simplex chronicus, chronic eczema, atopic dermatitis, and chronic lichen simplex are among the possible differential diagnoses. The beginning, length, and development of lesions, together with any related systemic symptoms, must be part of a comprehensive clinical history. Differentiating PN from these other disorders can be achieved through histopathological study of a biopsy.

The Methods Used in Clinical Examinations

Pay close attention to the location and shape of the lesions as you do a thorough clinical evaluation. The quantity, size, and color of the nodules, in addition to any indications of secondary infection, should be evaluated throughout the examination. The nodules' firmness and depth can be evaluated by palpation. Dermoscopy can help find alterations in the skin's surface or unusual vascular patterns.

Evaluations in Dermatology

To diagnose PN, a dermatologist must do a thorough skin examination and record the specifics of any lesions found. The nodules' surface features and blood vessels can be further assessed with dermoscopy. To further measure the severity of the condition and its impact on the patient's quality of life, standardized instruments like the Dermatology Life Quality Index (DLQI) and the Prurigo Activity Score (PAS) can be utilized.

Laboratory and Imaging Studies

While imaging tests aren't usually necessary to diagnose PN, they can help rule out other possible causes. To rule out systemic diseases that could be exacerbating the pruritus, a full blood count (CBC), testing for the liver and kidneys, and tests for the thyroid could be ordered in the lab. It is possible, depending on the patient's condition, that serological testing for infections and autoimmune illnesses is necessary.

Techniques for Biopsies

To rule out other possible causes and establish a diagnosis of PN, a skin biopsy is frequently required. To get a good sample of the epidermis, dermis, and underlying tissues, the biopsy needs to cover the entire skin's thickness. The dermis usually exhibits a mixed inflammatory infiltration, hyperkeratosis, and acanthosis upon histopathological investigation. The presence of eosinophils and cutaneous fibrosis can be observed.

Updates to Diagnostic Criteria

Clinical and histological findings should be considered together, according to new PN diagnostic criteria. Critical to the diagnosis is the appearance of nodular lesions, prolonged pruritus, and a supporting histological pattern. It is equally important to rule out other pruritic dermatoses using clinical and laboratory testing.

In-Depth Analysis and Case Studies

To better understand the many manifestations and approaches of PN management, case studies are a great resource. Consider the following instance: a middle-aged woman with a history of atopic dermatitis presents with numerous pruritic nodules on the extensor surfaces. This case highlights the need to include PN in the differential diagnosis. A comprehensive clinical evaluation, confirmation of the diagnosis through histopathology, and evaluation of possible systemic underlying diseases are all necessary for the interpretation of such cases. Case studies are useful for gaining a better knowledge of the condition and developing future management strategies based on treatment responses and patient outcomes.

Healthcare providers can better diagnose, manage, and care for patients with Prurigo Nodularis if they have a thorough awareness of these characteristics.

CHAPTER 5

METHODS FOR TREATMENT

Treatments Applied Topically

Treatment for prurigo nodularis (PN) typically begins with topical medications, particularly for mild to moderate instances. These treatments are designed to help decrease inflammation, soothe itching, and speed up the healing process of the skin.

1. **Corticosteroids**: Dermatologists frequently recommend topical corticosteroids to alleviate irritation and inflammation. They are available in different strengths, with the strongest ones being saved for the most extreme instances. But there are negative effects, like skin thinning, that can occur with long-term use.

2. Applying non-steroidal anti-inflammatory creams like tacrolimus or pimecrolimus, which are calcineurin inhibitors, to delicate areas like

the face or intertriginous zones can help alleviate inflammation. Without the negative effects of steroids, they aid in regulating the immunological response.

3. **Capsaicin Cream**: This pepper-derived topical can help reduce itching by desensitizing skin nerve endings. Consistent use is required, and you could feel some burning at first.

4. **Camphor and Menthol**: The cooling action of these substances might provide temporary relief from itching. These are common ingredients in topical anti-itch lotions sold at drugstores.

5. The anti-inflammatory and antipruritic characteristics of coal tar make it a useful tool in the fight against nodule formation. But it stinks and can be a pain to clean up afterward.

6. One of the most important things you can do to manage PN is to use a moisturizer. To keep the skin hydrated and in good condition and lessen the chances of more irritation and nodules, you can use barrier repair creams and emollients.

Medications Used Systemically

Systemic drugs could be needed when topical treatments don't cut it. These drugs target the root causes of PN from the inside out.

1. The main use of antihistamines is to alleviate itching, and there are two types: first-generation (sedating) and second-generation (non-sedating). In many cases, they serve as supplementary treatment.

2. Immunosuppressants are medications that lower inflammation and immune system activity. Examples of these include cyclosporine and methotrexate. Due to their possible negative effects, these are usually reserved for severe, refractory patients.

3. **Systemic Corticosteroids**: While oral corticosteroids may alleviate severe symptoms rapidly, they come with serious side effects like osteoporosis, hypertension, and diabetes, which limit their usage in the long run.

4. **Thalidomide**: **Thalidomide** is a well-known immunomodulatory drug that can cure PN. However, it should be taken with caution because of its teratogenic risk and other severe side effects.

5. **Antibiotics**: To eliminate the infection and let the skin heal, antibiotics may be needed if secondary bacterial infections are present.

6. To alleviate the PN-related neuropathic pain and itching, neuromodulators such as gabapentin and pregabalin are available.

The Many Forms of Phototherapy

One treatment option for PN is phototherapy, which uses UV light to cure skin disorders.

1. **UVB Phototherapy**: As a standard practice, narrowband ultraviolet B light (NB-UVB) penetrates the skin at appropriate wavelengths to alleviate inflammation.

2. **PUVA Therapy**: This method incorporates both ultraviolet A (UVA) radiation and psoralen, a photosensitizing drug. For more serious cases, doctors may prescribe PUVA, which is more powerful than UVB but comes with a longer list of potential adverse effects, such as premature skin aging and an increased chance of skin cancer.

3. **Excimer Laser**: This type of UVB therapy is aimed specifically at lesions, reducing the risk of damage to healthy skin in the surrounding area.

Psychological Support

Because PN is associated with substantial psychological suffering, such as anxiety and depression, as a result of persistent itching and visible skin lesions, psychological therapies are of the utmost importance.

1. Cognitive Behavioural Therapy (CBT): Patients with PN can benefit from CBT by learning to cope with the emotional toll of the condition and cutting back on behaviors like scratching that make it worse.

2. **Methods for Managing Stress**: Mindfulness, meditation, and relaxation exercises are some ways to manage stress, which is known to cause or exacerbate PN symptoms.

3. Patients suffering from PN may find it helpful to join a support group where they may receive emotional support and hear stories from others who understand what it's like to live with the disease.

4. Medication for underlying mental health issues: **Psychotropic Medications**: Antidepressants and anxiolytics are two examples of the kinds of medications that may be recommended.

Methods of Integrative Medicine

The goal of integrative medicine is to improve health by integrating conventional and complementary care.

1. **Acupuncture**: By inserting tiny needles into precise anatomical spots, acupuncture helps some people alleviate pain and irritation while restoring internal harmony.

2. **Herbal Remedies**: Some herbs, like as licorice root or chamomile, can be used orally or applied topically to alleviate PN symptoms because of their anti-inflammatory characteristics.

3. **Nutritional Therapy**: To promote skin health and decrease inflammation, eat a diet high in anti-inflammatory nutrients. These include foods like vitamins, antioxidants, and omega-3 fatty acids. If you want to keep inflammation at bay, it's best to stay away from processed meals and refined sugars.

4. Relaxation, better blood flow, and less stress are all potential benefits of mind-body techniques like qigong, yoga, and tai chi for those with PN.

It's Important to Think About When Having Surgery

After all other methods have been exhausted, or if the nodule is too large to respond to less intrusive treatments, surgical intervention may be considered.

1. **Cryotherapy**: This treatment uses liquid nitrogen to freeze the nodules, which shrinks them and stops them from itching.

2. **Laser Surgery**: By giving targeted and accurate treatment with minimal injury to surrounding tissue, lasers can be utilized to remove or reduce the size of nodules.

3. **Excision**: The nodules may need to be surgically removed in certain instances. This is usually seen as a last resort when all other treatments have failed, but it can offer quick relief.

New and Future Treatments

Investigations into PN are continuing, and several potential therapies are being considered.

1. Clinical trials for **Biologic Therapies** have revealed encouraging results, with monoclonal antibodies targeting specific components of the immune system, such as IL-4 receptor antagonist dupilumab and anti-IL-31 antibody nemolizumab.

2. A novel therapy option may be available in the form of tiny molecules called **Janus Kinase (JAK) Inhibitors**. These molecules block the signaling pathways that are involved in immune responses and inflammation.

3. **Medications that Block Neurokinin-1 Receptors**: These medications have been found to alleviate pruritus in people with PN by targeting the pathways that cause itching.

Strategies for Combination Therapy

The goal of combination therapy is to improve results by utilizing various treatment techniques in a coordinated fashion.

1. To address both the local and systemic components of an illness, it can be helpful to combine topical therapy with systemic drugs. This combination can provide more thorough relief.

2. By lowering inflammation and increasing the skin's receptivity to medicines, phototherapy can improve the effectiveness of topical treatments.

3. **Integrative Approaches**: Enhancing health and well-being can be achieved by integrating traditional treatments with integrative medical techniques.

Care Focused on the Individual

The hallmark of patient-centered care is an emphasis on personalization of care according to each patient's unique requirements and preferences.

1. Patients' opinions, interests, and concerns can be better considered when they are actively involved in making decisions (a practice known as "shared decision-making").

2. Improving results can be achieved by the use of personalized treatment programs that take into account each patient's unique symptoms, way of life, and reaction to prior therapies.

3. Comprehensive treatment that promotes overall well-being is achieved by a holistic approach that addresses the physical, psychological, and social components of PN.

Problems with Adherence and Compliance

Effective management of PN requires patients to follow their treatment plan to the letter.

1. **Education**: One way to increase adherence is to educate patients about their disease and why it's important to follow treatment instructions.

2. **Simplifying Regimens**: One way to improve adherence is to make treatment regimens simpler. This can be done by combining therapies or reducing the number of daily applications.

3. **Support Systems**: Patients are more likely to complete their treatment plans when they have access to healthcare specialists, reminders, and follow-up appointments.

4. **Addressing Barriers**: **Successful Management** requires identifying and addressing obstacles to adherence, such as side effects, prescription expense, or difficulties getting treatments.

Healthcare practitioners can better treat prurigo nodularis and improve patients' quality of life and overall results by gaining a thorough understanding of and attending to each of these components.

CHAPTER 6

KNOWLEDGE FOR PATIENTS AND THEIR OWN HEALTH CARE

Insight into the Diagnosis Process

Nodules or bumps that are extremely irritating are the hallmarks of Prurigo nodularis (PN), a skin ailment that can last for years. Excruciating itching is a common symptom of these nodules, which can vary in size from little papules to bigger masses and greatly affect a person's quality of life. Although the precise mechanism by which PN develops remains a mystery, researchers suspect that a combination of hereditary, environmental, and immune variables have a role.

Changes to One's Way of Life

You can effectively treat PN symptoms by making specific lifestyle alterations. Some examples are:

- **Refraining from Scratching:** It may be difficult, but try not to scratch the afflicted regions. Doing so will help avoid additional discomfort and infection.

- **Wear Loose Clothes:** To lessen skin friction and irritation, wear loose, breathable clothing.

To minimize flare-ups and alleviate itching, it is important to maintain optimal skin hygiene by regularly cleansing and moisturizing the skin.

A Guide to Skin Care

Effective skincare is essential for the management of PN. Here are a few pointers:

To avoid irritating the skin, use gentle, fragrance-free cleansers.

To protect the skin from drying up and becoming even itchier, use a moisturizer regularly.

The use of harsh soaps, detergents, and skincare products might aggravate sensitive skin, so it's best to avoid them.

Methods for Reducing Itch

Itching relief is an important part of PN treatment. Methods to alleviate itching encompass:

- **Cool Compresses:** You can get brief relief from itching by using cool, damp compresses on the areas that are affected.

To relieve inflammation and itching, your healthcare professional may recommend topical medicines or ointments.

- **Avoiding Triggers:** Figure out what makes your itching worse, including specific textiles, high temperatures, or stress, and stay away from those things.

Methods for De-Stressing

Illness symptoms associated with PN can be exacerbated by stress. Methods to alleviate tension encompass:

Relaxation and stress reduction are two benefits of the practices of mindfulness and meditation.

Exercising regularly has several health benefits, including improving mood and lowering stress.

For emotional support and coping mechanisms, **Seeking Support:** Consulting a therapist or becoming a member of a support group are good options.

Food Suggestions

Although changes to one's diet may not alleviate PN symptoms entirely, they may assist:

Foods High in Omega-3 Fatty Acids, Antioxidants, and Anti-Inflammatory Properties: Include seafood, fruits, vegetables, nuts, and other foods that fall into this category.

To maintain healthy skin and the body as a whole, it is important to drink enough water.

- **Removing Triggers:** Some people experience itching and irritation in response to specific meals, such as spicy foods or alcohol. A meal journal could help you pinpoint what sets off your symptoms.

Why Consistent Follow-ups Are Crucial

It is crucial to have regular check-ups with your doctor to track the development of PN and make any necessary adjustments to your treatment plan. Your healthcare practitioner will be able to review the effectiveness of your treatment, discuss any worries you may have, and have a look at your symptoms at these appointments.

Tracking Development

You and your doctor can make better judgments when you record your symptoms and how your treatment is going. Keep track of your symptoms, their onset and progression, and how your body reacts to treatment by keeping a journal or diary.

Activating Networks of Support

The emotional support, shared experiences, and coping mechanisms that can be gained from connecting with others who have PN or attending support groups are priceless. Some great places to find people to lean on in times of need are patient advocacy groups, online forums, and local support groups.

Supporting Others and Standing Up

Improving results and quality of life can be achieved through self-empowerment through education on PN, advocacy for one's needs, and active participation in one's treatment plan. Always ask questions, be vocal about your concerns, and keep up with the latest treatment alternatives by participating in shared decision-making with your healthcare team.

You can improve your overall health and effectively manage Prurigo Nodularis by learning about the disease, making lifestyle changes, using proper skin care, dealing with itching and stress, following dietary recommendations, making regular follow-ups a priority, monitoring your progress, connecting with support networks, and advocating for yourself.

CHAPTER 7

PSYCHOLOGICAL EFFECTS

Prurigo nodularis and Its Mental Impact

Nodules that are extremely irritating are the hallmark of Prurigo nodularis (PN), a skin ailment that can last for years. Constant itching and scratching have a devastating effect on sufferers' mental health. Discomfort, hopelessness, and frustration are common emotions that can result from living with chronic pain. The long-term effects of a chronic illness on a person's mental and emotional well-being can lead to a decline in their quality of life. Because the skin lesions are so obvious, patients may feel even more self-conscious about their bodies and develop a poor self-image as a result.

Relationships Between Depression and Anxiety

A great deal of mental anguish can result from PN's chronic itching and the development of nodules. The constant pain and shame that come with the disease make many sufferers anxious and depressed. Sleep disruptions and the social isolation that many patients endure compound the psychological burden. The importance of including complete mental health assistance in the treatment plan for PN is highlighted by studies that show higher rates of anxiety and depression in this population compared to the general population.

Problems With Sleeping

For those with PN, sleep disruptions are a big deal. The severe itching usually gets worse at night, which makes it hard to fall asleep and wakes you up many times during the night. Irritability, anxiety, and sadness are already negatively affecting mental health, and chronic sleep loss can make these worse. Antihistamines, cognitive behavioral therapy for insomnia, and excellent sleep hygiene habits are all ways to improve the quality of sleep, which is important for the management of PN.

Isolation and Social Stigma

People may feel stigmatized and alone if they have PN or another visible skin disorder. Some patients may withdraw from social activities and interactions due to feelings of self-consciousness regarding their looks. Loneliness and mental health problems like anxiety and depression can worsen in such an isolated environment. To lessen the social stigma and build a community of support for people living with PN, public awareness initiatives and support groups are vital.

Dealing with Adversity

To deal with the mental toll that PN takes, coping skills are crucial. Some examples of these methods are relaxation exercises, mindfulness practices, and cognitive-behavioral approaches. To alleviate the itching and boost mood, it can be helpful to encourage people to participate in things they enjoy. The best way for patients to deal with the emotional toll that a sickness can take is to surround themselves with supportive people, whether that's family, friends, or healthcare providers.

Interventions for Treatment

Physical symptoms and the emotional pain that goes along with them should be treated together in PN treatment plans. Topical and systemic pharmacological therapy are available for the reduction of inflammation and itching. Patients can learn to control their anxiety, sadness, and stress with the help of psychological therapies like CBT and ACT. A more comprehensive approach to treatment can be achieved by combining dermatological care with mental health treatments.

Support for Family and Carers

When it comes to helping people with PN, family and carers are crucial. By learning more about the illness, they will be better able to empathize with the patient and provide appropriate assistance. Feeling less alone and more supported is possible when family members are encouraged to communicate openly with one another. Maintaining good mental health is essential for carers; they should reach out for help and take breaks when they need them to avoid burnout.

Meeting Mental Health Requirements

Recognizing the psychological impact of PN and offering suitable assistance are essential in addressing the emotional needs of patients with the illness. Screenings, therapy, and support groups for mental health issues should be part of this routine. Medical professionals should show empathy and compassion by listening to and acknowledging their patients' stories and worries. The quality of life for people with PN can be greatly improved by incorporating psychological assistance into their treatment programs.

Approaches to Mental Health that Integrate

When it comes to mental health, integrative methods take a more comprehensive approach by combining traditional medical care with complementary therapies. Acupuncture, yoga, meditation, and nutritional counseling are some of the techniques that can help with general health and mental wellness. Patients with PN can benefit from stress management, symptom reduction, and improved coping abilities when these strategies are part of their treatment strategy.

Stories of Resilience and Triumph

People dealing with PN can offer hope and encouragement to others going through tough times by sharing their experiences of resilience and recovery. It could be empowering to hear of patients' successes in symptom management, quality of life enhancement, and psychological hurdles overcoming. The significance of a holistic approach to treatment, encompassing both physical and mental health resources, may be demonstrated through these accounts. People living with PN can have a more positive view if resilience is promoted through patient education, support networks, and positive reinforcement.

In conclusion, Prurigo Nodularis has far-reaching and complex psychological effects that manifest in many ways throughout a patient's life. Efficacious medical care, psychological support, and methods to enhance social and emotional health are all necessary to address this impact. Patients with PN might greatly benefit from healthcare practitioners who acknowledge and treat the mental health issues that come with the condition.

CHAPTER 8

INVESTIGATING AND DEVELOPING NEW TECHNOLOGIES

Today's Popular Areas of Study

1. **Understanding Pathophysiology**:

Neurogenic inflammation, immunological dysregulation, and the function of sensory nerves in persistent itching are the subject of present-day investigations into the pathophysiology of Prurigo nodularis (PN).

2. To properly categorize PN subgroups and facilitate focused treatment options, researchers are emphasizing comprehensive phenotyping as part of the clinical characterization process.

3. Psychological Factors: Investigating the relationship between mental health issues, such

as stress and anxiety, and PN flare-ups, to develop comprehensive approaches to treatment.

4. To enhance worldwide management guidelines, researchers in the field of global epidemiology are studying geographical variations in the prevalence of PN, risk factors, and healthcare inequities.

The Role of Biomarkers and Genetics

1. Researchers are finding genetic variations linked to PN vulnerability, which could explain familial clustering and other hereditary variables.

2. **Biomarker Discovery**: To help in diagnosis, disease monitoring, and therapy response prediction, researchers are investigating biomarkers in blood, skin, and neuroimaging.

New Discoveries in Immunology

1. **Inflammatory Pathways**: **Targeting Immunomodulatory Therapies** by studying immune-mediated pathways including Th1/Th2

balance, cytokine profiles, and mast cell activation.

2. Discovering new autoimmune-targeted therapeutics requires first understanding autoimmune pathways and how they contribute to PN development.

Emerging Targeted Treatments

1. The effectiveness of neurokinin receptor antagonists in lowering lesion burden and halting the itch-scratch cycle is being evaluated in trials.

2. Investigating the use of monoclonal antibodies to target specific cytokines or immune cells that are involved in the pathophysiology of PN.

3. **Small Molecule Inhibitors**: Designing and developing small molecule inhibitors to control itch perception and inflammation by targeting pruritogenic receptors or enzymes.

Strategies for Repurposing Drugs

1.   Utilising   **Present   Dermatological Medications**: Applying immunomodulatory and anti-inflammatory characteristics of medications such as antihistamines, topical corticosteroids, and calcineurin inhibitors to the management of PN.

2. The effectiveness of neuropharmaceuticals, including gabapentinoids and tricyclic antidepressants, in modulating itching sensations.

Uses of Artificial Intelligence

1. **Diagnostic Algorithms**: Applying ML algorithms to clinical, histological, and imaging data for precise PN diagnosis.

2. Utilising artificial intelligence to forecast how a person will react to a treatment, improve therapy selection, and lessen side effects is known as **Treatment Response Prediction**.

Trials Focused on Patients

1. **Patient Reported Outcomes (PROs)**: Using PROs in clinical studies to measure changes in treatment effectiveness, intensity of symptoms, and quality of life as perceived by the patients themselves.

2. The use of telemedicine and other digital health platforms to conduct trials virtually has the potential to increase patient engagement, decrease trial load, and facilitate distant monitoring.

Projects that Involve Collaboration

1. To expedite PN research, **international consortia** brings together research institutes, businesses, and patient advocacy organizations to pool resources, knowledge, and data.

2. To address PN from multiple angles and create all-encompassing treatment plans, dermatologists, immunologists, neurologists, and

psychologists should work together as multi-disciplinary teams.

Financing & Subsidies

1. Funding for fundamental research, clinical trials, and translational studies can be obtained through **Public-Private Partnerships**, which involve partnering with pharmaceutical corporations, philanthropic organizations, and government bodies.

2. **Early Career Research Grants**: Supporting the pursuit of novel PN research by promising young scientists via fellowships and grants.

Prurigo nodularis research: where we go from here

1. Precision medicine is making strides towards tailoring treatment plans to each patient by analyzing their genetic makeup, biomarker patterns, and other unique characteristics.

2. **Regenerative Therapies**: Looking into ways to manage PN in the long run using stem cell therapies, tissue engineering, and gene editing.

3. **Digital Health Integration**: For early intervention methods, self-management, and continuous PN monitoring, integrating wearable devices, digital biomarkers, and AI-driven platforms is essential.

This all-inclusive resource details recent and continuing research on Prurigo Nodularis, a difficult dermatological illness, and how interdisciplinary innovation is needed to better understand, treat, and eventually prevent it.

CHAPTER 9

VIEWS AND OBSTACLES ON A GLOBAL SCALE

Healthcare Access on a Global Scale

There is a huge global disparity in the availability of treatment for Prurigo nodularis (PN). Patients in industrialized nations typically have less trouble gaining access to dermatologists and more sophisticated therapies like biologics and phototherapy. In contrast, dermatologists are in short supply, healthcare facilities are inadequate, and budgetary restrictions mean that patients in underdeveloped nations often go without the specialized treatment they need. Timely diagnosis and successful treatment might also be impeded by geographical constraints and restricted pharmaceutical availability. International healthcare collaborations, telemedicine, and mobile clinics are some of the ways that people are working to enhance access so that underprivileged communities can get the treatment they need.

Healthcare Inequalities

There is a significant racial/ethnic/geographic gap in healthcare access and quality of care for PNs. Delays in diagnosis and less thorough care are experienced by minority communities and those with lower socioeconomic status, according to studies. The disease may proceed more rapidly and the quality of life may decrease as a result. A combination of community engagement programs, improved financing for public health efforts aimed at underprivileged communities, and legislative changes to guarantee equal healthcare access are necessary to address these gaps.

Cultural Factors Affecting Health Care

When it comes to PN therapy, cultural attitudes and traditions matter a great deal. Delays in receiving effective care may occur in some cultures because traditional medicines and alternative medicine are valued more highly than contemporary therapies. To provide patient-centered care and increase treatment adherence, healthcare providers must understand cultural backgrounds. To make sure that patients' treatments are in keeping with their beliefs and practices while still following medical guidelines, it is important to use culturally sensitive communication and teaching tactics to increase patient trust and participation.

The Consequences of Health Policy

The administration of PN is greatly influenced by health policies. Subsidized medicine programs and more financing for dermatological research are examples of policies that encourage fair access to healthcare and can greatly enhance patient outcomes. Also, policies should be put in place to increase the availability of dermatologists, especially in underserved areas. Reducing the financial strain on patients and healthcare systems can also be achieved by advocating for measures that improve insurance coverage and address the high cost of PN treatments.

Prurigo nodularin's financial impact

Patients and healthcare systems are financially burdened by PN. Expenses associated with doctor visits, prescription drugs, and hospital stays are examples of direct costs. Negative effects on mental health, decreased ability to work, and lost productivity are examples of indirect expenses associated with chronic illness. The necessity for more efficient use of healthcare funds and more cost-effective treatment methods is brought to light by the quantification of this burden. Research and programs to lessen the monetary toll of PN on people and society can be bolstered by economic evaluations, which can influence governmental decisions.

Efforts to Advocate

To bring attention to PN and influence policy changes, advocacy actions are vital. To educate the public, fund research, and advocate for better healthcare legislation, patient advocacy groups and professional organizations are crucial. Greater public knowledge of PN, higher quality patient treatment, and more financing for PN research are all possible outcomes of these endeavors. To ensure a cohesive approach to addressing the difficulties of PN, effective lobbying frequently entails collaboration with stakeholders, including healthcare providers, researchers, and politicians.

Collaborations on a Global Scale

To further our understanding and treatment of PN, international cooperation is crucial. Advancements in disease processes, treatment options, and epidemiology can be made through collaborative research endeavors. When people from different countries work together, it becomes much easier to combat PN on a global scale, especially in places where resources are scarce. By working together, groups like the World Health Organisation (WHO) and international dermatology societies can standardize treatment protocols and spread awareness of best practices across the globe.

Education and Training Requirements

Improved education and training for healthcare providers on PN is urgently required. All members of the healthcare team, including primary care physicians, dermatologists, and others, need up-to-date training on the most recent diagnostic tools, treatment methods, and management techniques. Workshops, online courses, and continuing medical education (CME) programs can assist in filling in knowledge gaps. Furthermore, future healthcare providers will be adequately educated to address this problem by including PN education in medical school curricula.

Innovations in Telemedicine

For areas without easy access to dermatologists, telemedicine has been an invaluable resource for PN management. Patients in rural locations can now access specialized dermatological care through teledermatology, which eliminates the need for in-person consultations by allowing for remote diagnosis and treatment planning. Technology advancements, such as teleconsultation platforms and mobile health apps, allow for better monitoring and communication between patients and doctors, which in turn improves treatment adherence and results. To fully harness the power of telemedicine in PN care, however, obstacles like internet accessibility and regulatory concerns must be resolved.

Dealing with the Worldwide Effects

A holistic strategy that prioritizes expanding access to care, decreasing healthcare disparities, and promoting international cooperation is necessary to address the worldwide burden of PN. All patients, regardless of their financial situation or where they live, should have access to good therapies, and public health campaigns should aim to raise awareness and encourage early diagnosis. Prioritizing financing for PN research and supporting worldwide efforts to standardize care procedures should be global health policy priorities. The worldwide community can help alleviate PN and enhance the lives of people impacted by it by working together in an inclusive and coordinated manner.

CHAPTER 10

GIVING BACK TO THE PRURIGO NODULARIS PEOPLE

Rights and Responsibilities of Patients

The Rights of Patients:

1. **Access to Care:** All patients have the entitlement to prompt and suitable medical attention, which encompasses diagnostic procedures and therapies tailored to Prurigo nodularis (PN).

2. To ensure that patients can make well-informed decisions about their care, it is essential that they receive complete and accurate information about their disease, treatment options, risks, and benefits.

3. Healthcare providers have a responsibility to safeguard their patients' private information by

keeping their medical records and other personal data secure.

4. **Participation in Care:** Patients are entitled to inquire about their care and take an active role in developing their treatment plans.

5. Every patient has the right to get care that does not favor one group over another, regardless of their gender, age, handicap, or financial background.

What the Patient Must Do

1. The patient must be forthright and honest with their healthcare professionals regarding their current condition, any symptoms they may be experiencing, and any relevant medical history.

2. **Treatment Compliance:** To properly manage PN, it is essential to follow the recommended treatment programs and show up for scheduled visits.

3. **Provider Respect:** Patients are expected to show the utmost deference and politeness towards healthcare providers and personnel.

4. **Recognising Limitations:** Acknowledging that healthcare practitioners are limited in their ability to deliver optimal care due to limitations in medical knowledge and available resources.

5. If patients have questions about their diagnosis or treatment, they should talk to their doctors to get their questions answered.

Groups and Tools for Advocacy

Big Names in Advocacy:

1. **National Eczema Association (NEA):** The NEA is a great resource for anyone dealing with eczema or a similar condition, such as PN, by providing information, education, and support.

2. **The American Skin Association (ASA):** Provides support for PN and other skin disorders

through advocacy, education, and research funding.

3. International organizations aiming to better the lives of persons affected by dermatological problems are supported by **Global Skin**, an alliance that spans the globe.

What We Have to Offer:

1. **Educational Resources**: Slideshows, articles, and brochures regarding PN signs, therapies, and ways to handle the condition.

2. Peer support groups, patient forums, and helplines are all ways that people can get in touch with PN.

3. Assistance with Payment: **Financial Assistance:** Details on grants, insurance navigating, and programs that provide financial aid to assist with the cost of treatment.

Community Support Groups

Why Support Groups Are Crucial:

Assists patients in overcoming feelings of loneliness by creating a secure environment in which they may open up about their struggles.

- **Real-World Guidance:** Community members can share their experiences with symptom management, coping mechanisms, and understanding how to use healthcare resources.

- **Empowerment and Advocacy:** Many support groups work to increase patient rights by speaking out against injustice and bringing attention to important issues.

Recognising a Community of Support:

PN-specific groups are commonly hosted on online platforms such as Facebook, Reddit, and specialized forums.

- **Local Chapters:** A large number of national organizations have associated groups that meet and host events on a more local level.

Healthcare Provider Referrals: Primary care physicians and dermatologists are good resources for finding trustworthy support groups.

Public Education Initiatives

Awareness campaigns serve a purpose:

- **Raise Awareness:** Get the word out about PN, its signs, and the difficulties endured by individuals impacted.

- **Stimulate Prompt Medical Attention:** Urge those who are suffering symptoms to consult a doctor as soon as possible.

- **Promote Understanding:** Assist the general public in comprehending the effects of PN on day-to-day living, thus decreasing prejudice and misunderstandings.

Strategies for a Fruitful Campaign

1. Utilising social media sites like Facebook, Instagram, and Twitter to disseminate information about patients, research, and awareness activities.

2. **Public Events:** Inviting the public and media through the planning of walks, lectures, and health fairs.

3. **Collaborations:** Working together with other health organizations, celebrities, and influencers to increase exposure.

Advocating for Policies

Policy Advocacy Objectives:

Improve Access to Care: Advocate for regulations that make it easier for people with PN to get the care they need, including specialists and therapies.

- **Seek More Money for Research:** Push for more funding for PN research from both the public and commercial sectors.

- In the realm of insurance, it is important to strive for policies that provide full coverage of PN treatments and prescriptions.

Where You Can Make a Difference:

1. **Reach Out to Legislators:** Communicate with your lawmakers on PN matters by writing letters, sending emails, or setting up meetings.

2. **Join Advocacy Groups:** Take part in events hosted by groups whose mission is to raise awareness about skin diseases and other chronic illnesses.

3. **Communicating with the Public:** Take part in public discussions and hearings regarding healthcare policies that impact people undergoing dermatological.

Opportunities to Participate in Research

Why Research Is Crucial:

Participation in clinical trials can result in the development of novel and more effective treatments for PN, which is an advancement in treatment.

- **Understanding the Disease:** To develop more effective management options, research is needed to understand the disease and its mechanisms.

- **Empowering Patients:** Taking part in research gives patients a voice in how science is done and gives them the chance to use innovative treatments.

How Can I Take Part?

1. Patients can find ongoing trials to participate in on websites like ClinicalTrials.gov.

2. Participation in patient registries allows for the collection of useful information on PN by researchers.

3. Taking part in studies and surveys run by academic institutions, such as surveys and observational studies.

Education for Healthcare Providers

Restaurant Owners:

- **Continuing Medical Education (CME)**: Suggest that primary care doctors and dermatologists take PN-focused CME courses.

- **Educational Events:** Host or participate in seminars and workshops that cover the most recent research and practices in PN diagnosis and treatment.

- **Resources and Literature:** Inform healthcare providers about PN breakthroughs by distributing thorough guidelines and research updates.

Educational Focus Areas:

1. The ability to recognize the symptoms of PN is crucial for prompt and correct diagnosis.

2. The treatment options for PN are currently being reviewed, including both established and new medicines.

3. Guidelines for having open and honest conversations about PN with patients, listening to their concerns, and including them in treatment decisions (**Patient Communication**).

Prurigo nodularis and technology

Innovations in Technology:

- **Telemedicine:** People in rural locations, in particular, can benefit from virtual consultations with professionals thanks to telemedicine.

- **Mobile Apps:** Applications made to monitor symptoms, keep track of when to take medication, and communicate this information to healthcare professionals.

Wearable Devices: Tools for keeping tabs on skin health, which aid in the control of related symptoms and events.

What are the advantages?

Technology lowers obstacles to accessing healthcare providers and specialists, leading to **Improved Access to Care**.

The condition can be effectively managed with the help of continuous monitoring devices, which provide enhanced monitoring.

- **Patient Engagement:** Patients are encouraged to actively participate in their own care and treatment adherence through the use of apps and online platforms.

Patient and Carer Testimonies

The Influence of Narratives:

- **Awareness and Education:** Sharing personal narratives about PN brings PN to a more human level and brings attention to the difficulties that patients and carers encounter daily.

- **Community Building:** When patients and carers talk to each other about their experiences, it helps to create a feeling of belonging and support.

- **Inspiration and Hope:** Individuals who are newly diagnosed or battling with PN can find inspiration and hope in hearing about the experiences of others.

Shared Media Platforms:

Ensure that patients have a personal blog or video blog where they can document their experiences and share their stories.

- **Social Media Campaigns**: Sites where users may connect and share tales, such as Instagram and Facebook.

Advocacy Group Websites: To bring attention to the issue and gather support, numerous advocacy groups showcase patient stories on their websites.

Building a Hopeful Future

A Look Towards the Future:

- **Research Towards a Cure and Improved therapies:** Ongoing efforts to discover a cure and develop better therapies for PN.

- **Comprehensive Care:** Methods for the holistic management of PN that take into account the patient's emotional, mental, and physical well-being.

Ensuring that all patients, irrespective of their location or socioeconomic situation, have access to the care and services they need is the goal of **Universal Access**.

How to Reach This Goal:

1. Participate in and contribute to research projects centered on PN to **Support Research**.

2. **Get the Word Out:** Launch Initiatives to Inform the General People and Government Officials About PN.

3. **Speak Out for Patients:** Push for legislative reforms that enhance the standard of living for individuals afflicted by PN.

4. Create safe spaces for patients and carers to meet and support one another; this will help foster a community of care.

Finally, there is no one-size-fits-all solution to empowering the Prurigo Nodularis community. We must all work together to protect patients' rights, disseminate information, build stronger communities, take part in scientific studies, and make the most of available technological resources. A future where PN patients receive the treatment and support they need can be ours through policy advocacy and awareness-raising. This will lead to better outcomes and a higher quality of life for these patients.